The Complete Renal Diet Cookbook 2021

-An Easy to Follow Guide to Drastically Reduce Chances of Kidney Disease with Quick and Delicious Recipes-

[Simona Malcom]

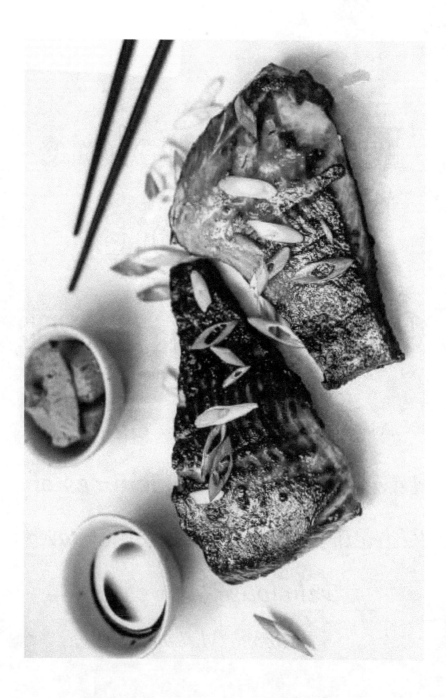

Table Of Content

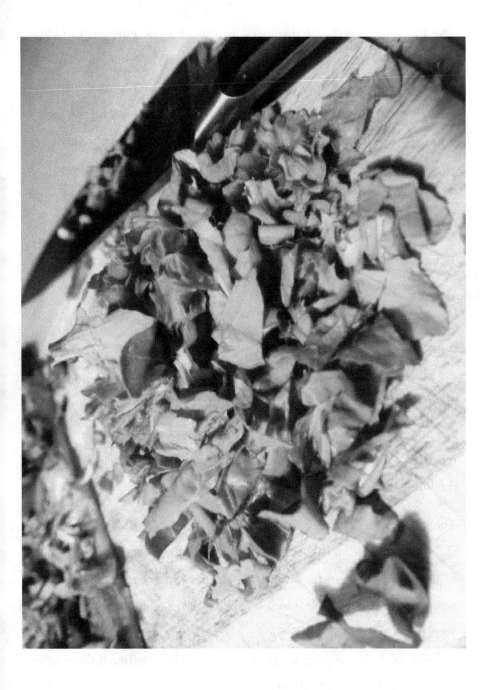

The following Book is reproduced below with the goal of providing information that is as accurate and reliable as possible. Regardless, purchasing this Book can be seen as consent to the fact that both the publisher and the author of this book are in no way experts on the topics discussed within and that any recommendations or suggestions that are made herein are for entertainment purposes only. Professionals should be consulted as needed prior to undertaking any of the action endorsed herein.

This declaration is deemed fair and valid by both the American Bar Association and the Committee of Publishers Association and is legally binding throughout the United States.

Furthermore, the transmission, duplication, or reproduction of any of the following work including specific information will be considered an illegal act irrespective of if it is done electronically or in print. This extends to creating a secondary or tertiary copy of the work or a recorded copy and is only allowed with the express written consent from the Publisher. All additional right reserved.

The information in the following pages is broadly considered a truthful and accurate account of facts and as such, any inattention, use, or misuse of the information in question by the reader will render any resulting actions solely under their purview. There are no scenarios in which the publisher or the original author of this work can be in any fashion deemed liable for any hardship or damages that may befall them after undertaking information described herein.

Additionally, the information in the following pages is intended only for informational purposes and should thus be thought of as universal. As befitting its nature, it is presented without assurance regarding its prolonged validity or interim quality. Trademarks that are mentioned are done without written consent and can in no way be considered an endorsement from the trademark holder.

CHAPTER 1: Introduction

Human health hangs in a complete balance when all of its interconnected bodily mechanisms function properly in perfect sync. Without its major organs working normally, the body soon suffers indelible damage. Kidney malfunction is one such example, and it is not just the entire water balance that is disturbed by the kidney disease, but a number of other diseases also emerge due to this problem.

Kidney diseases are progressive, meaning that they can ultimately lead to permanent kidney damage if left unchecked and uncontrolled. That is why it is essential to control and manage the disease and halt its progress, which can be done through medicinal and natural means. While medicines can guarantee only thirty percent of the cure, a change of lifestyle and diet can prove miraculous with their seventy percent guaranteed results. A kidney-friendly diet and lifestyle not only saves the kidneys from excess minerals, but it also aids medicines to work actively. Treatment without a good diet, hence, proves to be useless. In this renal diet cookbook, we shall bring out the basic facts about kidney diseases, their symptoms, causes, and diagnosis. This preliminary introduction can help the readers understand the problem clearly; then, we shall discuss the role of renal diet and kidney-friendly lifestyle in curbing the diseases. It's not just that the book also contains a range of delicious renal diet recipes, which will guarantee luscious flavors and good health.

Despite their tiny size, the kidneys perform a number of functions, which are vital for the body to be able to function healthily.

These include:

- Filtering excess fluids and waste from the blood.

- Creating the enzyme known as renin, which regulates blood pressure.

- Ensuring bone marrow creates red blood cells.

- Controlling calcium and phosphorus levels through absorption and excretion.

Unfortunately, when kidney disease reaches a chronic stage, these functions start to stop working. However, with the right treatment and lifestyle, it is possible to manage symptoms and continue living well. This is even more applicable in the earlier stages of the disease. Tactlessly, 10% of all adults over the age of 20 will experience some form of kidney disease in their lifetime. There are a variety of different treatments for kidney disease, which depend on the cause of the disease.

According to international stats, kidney (or renal) diseases are affecting around 14% of the adult population. In the US, approx. 661.000 Americans suffer from kidney dysfunction. Out of these patients, 468.000 proceed to dialysis treatment, and the rest have one active kidney transplant.

The high quantities of diabetes and heart illness are also related to kidney dysfunction, and sometimes one condition, for example, diabetes, may prompt the other.

With such a significant number of high rates, possibly the best course of treatment is the contravention of dialysis, making people depend upon clinical and crisis facility meds in any occasion multiple times every week. In this manner, if your kidney has just given a few indications of brokenness, you can forestall dialysis through an eating routine, something that we will talk about in this book.

CHAPTER 2: Kidney disease

What is Kidney Disease?

A kidney disease diagnosis implies that the kidneys are either dysfunctional, under-functioning, or damaged and cannot filter out toxins and metabolic waste on their own. Our systems need our kidneys for a waste filtering process. However, when kidney damage occurs, the system is piled up with damaging waste that cannot expel through other means. As a result, inflammatory responses emerge, and you have a much higher chance of developing chronic and serious health disorders like diabetes or heart failure, which can even be fatal in extreme cases.

There are two main types of kidney disease, based on their cause and time duration:

● A sudden and unexpected kidney damage/acute kidney injury (AKI) as a result of an accident or surgery side effects, which usually lasts for a short period of time.

● Chronic and progressive kidney dysfunction (CKD). As its name suggests, this is a chronic condition with multiple progressive stages that lead ultimately to permanent kidney damage. There are approx. 5 stages of the disorder, and during the last and final stage, the patient will need dialysis or a kidney transplant to survive. This final stage is also known in the medical glossary as End-Stage-Renal Disease (ESRD).

There are higher than normal amounts of a certain protein called Arbutin in the urine during all kidney dysfunction stages, which can be confirmed by urine tests for diagnosing renal disease. This condition is known scientifically as Proteinuria. Doctors may also perform blood tests and/or image screening tests to pinpoint a problem with the kidneys and develop a diagnosis.

Causes of Kidney Disease?

There are many causes of kidney disease, including physical injury or disorders that can damage the kidneys, but the two leading causes of kidney disease are diabetes and high blood pressure. These underlying conditions also put people at risk for developing cardiovascular disease. Early treatment may not only slow down the progression of the disease, but also reduce your risk of developing heart disease or stroke.

Kidney disease can affect anyone at any age. African Americans, Hispanics, and American Indians are at increased risk for kidney failure because these groups have a greater prevalence of diabetes and high blood pressure.

Uncontrolled diabetes is the leading cause of kidney disease. Diabetes can damage the kidneys and cause them to fail.

The second leading cause of kidney disease is high blood pressure, also known as hypertension. One in three Americans is at risk for kidney disease because of hypertension. Although there is no cure for hypertension, certain medications, a low-sodium diet, and physical activity can lower blood pressure.

The kidneys help manage blood pressure, but when blood pressure is high, the heart has to work overtime at pumping blood. High blood pressure can damage the blood vessels in the kidneys, reducing their ability to work efficiently. When the force of blood flow is high, blood vessels start to stretch so the blood can flow more easily. The stretching and scarring weaken the blood vessels throughout the entire body, including the kidneys. When the kidneys' blood vessels are injured, they may not remove the waste and extra fluid from the body, creating a dangerous cycle because the extra fluid in the blood vessels can increase blood pressure even more.

Cardiovascular disease is the leading cause of death in the United States. When kidney disease occurs, that process can be affected, and the risk of developing heart disease becomes greater. Cardiovascular disease is an umbrella term used to describe conditions that may damage the heart and blood vessels, including coronary artery disease, heart attack, heart failure, atherosclerosis, and high blood pressure. Complications from a renal disease may develop and can lead to heart disease.

With diabetes, excess blood sugar remains in the bloodstream. The high blood sugar levels can damage the blood vessels in the kidneys and elsewhere in the body. And since high blood pressure is a complication from diabetes, the extra pressure can weaken the walls of the blood vessels, which can lead to a heart attack or stroke.

Other conditions, such as drug abuse and certain autoimmune diseases, can also cause injury to the kidneys. In fact, every drug we put into our body has to pass through the kidneys for filtration. If the drug is not taken following a healthcare provider's instructions, or if it is an illegal substance such as heroin, cocaine, or ecstasy, it can cause injury to the kidneys by raising the blood pressure, also increasing the risk of a stroke, heart failure, and even death.

An autoimmune disease is one in which the immune system, designed to protect the body from illness, sees the body as an invader and attacks its own systems, including the kidneys. Some forms of lupus, for example, attack the kidneys. Another autoimmune disease that can lead to kidney failure is Goodpasture syndrome, a group of conditions that affect the kidneys and the lungs. The damage to the kidneys from autoimmune diseases can lead to chronic kidney disease and kidney failure.

Symptoms of Kidney Disease?

Some people in the early stages of kidney disease may not even show any symptoms. If you suffer from diabetes or high blood pressure, it is important to manage it early on in order to protect your kidneys. Although kidney failure occurs over the course of many years, you may not show any signs until kidney disease or failure has occurred.

When the kidneys are damaged, wastes and toxins can build up in the body because the kidneys cannot filter them as effectively. Once this buildup begins, you may start to feel sick and experience some of the following symptoms:

- Anemia (low red blood cell count)
- Blood in urine
- Bone pain
- Difficulty concentrating
- Difficulty sleeping
- Dry and itchy skin
- Muscle cramps (especially in the legs)
- Nausea
- Poor appetite
- Swelling in feet and ankles
- Tiredness
- Weakness
- Weight loss

Fortunately, once treatment for kidney disease begins, especially if caught in the early stages, symptoms tend to lessen, and general health will begin to improve.

Diagnosis Tests

Besides identifying the symptoms of kidney disease, there are other better and more accurate ways to confirm the extent of loss of renal function. There are mainly two important diagnostic tests:

1. Urine Test

The urine test clearly states all the renal problems. The urine is the waste product of the kidney. When there is a loss of filtration or any hindrance to the kidneys, the urine sample will indicate it through the number of excretory products present in it. The severe stages of chronic disease show some amount of protein and blood in the urine. Do not rely on self-tests; visit an authentic clinic for these tests.

2. Blood Pressure and Blood Test

Another good way to check for renal disease is to test the blood and its composition. A high amount of creatinine and other waste products in the blood clearly indicates that the kidneys are not functioning properly. Blood pressure can also be indicative of renal disease. When the water balance in the body is disturbed, it may cause high blood pressure. Hypertension can both be the cause and symptom of kidney disease and, therefore, should be taken seriously.

Treatment

The best way to manage CKD is to be an active participant in your treatment program, regardless of your stage of renal disease. Proper treatment involves a combination of working with a healthcare team, adhering to a renal diet, and making healthy lifestyle decisions. These can all have a profoundly positive effect on your kidney disease—especially watching how you eat.

Working with Your Healthcare Team

When you have kidney disease, working in partnership with your healthcare team can be extremely important in your treatment program as well as being personally empowering. Regularly meeting with your physician or healthcare team can arm you with resources and information that help you make informed decisions regarding your treatment needs and provide you with a much-needed opportunity to vent, share information, get advice, and receive support in effectively managing this illness.

Adhering to a Renal Diet

The heart of this book is the renal diet. Sticking to this diet can make a huge difference in your health and vitality. Like any change, following the diet may not be easy at first. Important changes to your diet, particularly early on, can possibly prevent the need for dialysis. These changes include limiting salt, eating a low-protein diet, reducing fat intake, and getting enough calories if you need to lose weight. Be honest with yourself first and foremost—learn what you need, and consider your personal goals and obstacles. Start by making small changes. It is okay to have some slip-ups—we all do. With guidance and support, these small changes will become habits of your promising new lifestyle. In no time, you will begin taking control of your diet and health.

Making Healthy Lifestyle Decisions

Lifestyle choices play a crucial part in our health, especially when it comes to helping regulate kidney disease. Lifestyle choices such as allotting time for physical activity, getting enough sleep, managing weight, reducing stress, and limiting smoking and alcohol will help you take control of your overall health, making it easier to manage your kidney disease. Follow this simple formula: Keep toxins out of your body as much as you can, and build up your immune system with a good balance of exercise, relaxation, and sleep.

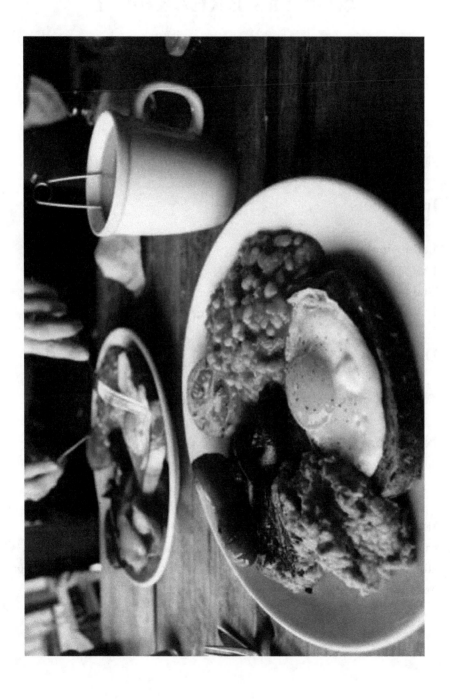

CHAPTER 3: **BREAKFAST**

Salmon Bagel

Prep:5 mins
Cook:5 mins
Servings:1

Ingredients

1 slice whole-grain bread toasted
1 ½ ounces sliced smoked salmon
2 tablespoons reduced-fat cream cheese softened
1/4 teaspoon everything bagel seasoning

Directions
1
Top toast with cream cheese, salmon and seasoning.

Nutrition
Serving Size: 1 Slice
:

181 calories; protein 13.7g; carbohydrates 13.9g; dietary fiber 2g;
sugars 3.4g; fat 7.6g; saturated fat 3.4g; cholesterol 26mg; vitamin a iu
202.9IU; vitamin c 0.1mg; folate 26.4mcg; calcium 79.3mg; iron 1.1mg;
magnesium 31.4mg; potassium 212.7mg; sodium 589.6mg.

Egg Whites Cups

Prep: 5 Mins
Cook: 5 Mins
Servings: 4

Ingredients

for 6 servings
1 roma tomato, 11 calories
2 cups egg white(480 mL), 250 calories
1 roma tomato, 11 calories
salt, to taste, 0 calories
2 cups spinach(60 g), 14 calories
½ teaspoon pepper, 0 calories

Directions

Preheat the oven to 350°F.
Lightly grease a muffin tin.
Then divide equally the spinach across 6 cups.
Dice the tomato, then fill the cups with the tomato and egg whites.
Season with salt and pepper.
Bake for 15 minutes, or until the whites have set.
Serve hot.
Enjoy!

Nutritions:

Fat 9g
Carbs 1g
Fiber 0g
Sugar 0g
Protein 12g

Chinese Stir – Fried Tomatoes Eggs

Prep:10 mins
Cook:5 mins
Servings:3

Ingredients

6 eggs, beaten
2 green onions, thinly sliced
4 ripe tomatoes, sliced into wedges
2 tablespoons avocado oil

Directions

Heat 1 tablespoon avocado oil in a wok or skillet over medium heat. Cook and stir eggs in the hot oil until mostly cooked through, 1 minute. Transfer eggs to a plate.

Pour remaining 1 tablespoon avocado oil into wok; cook and stir tomatoes until liquid has mostly evaporated, about 3 minutes. Return eggs to wok and add green onions; cook and stir until eggs are fully cooked, about 30 seconds.

Nutrition

:

264 calories
protein 14.5g
carbohydrates 9.2g
fat 19.7g
cholesterol 372mg
sodium 151.5mg

Sun Dried Tomato Frittata

Prep:20 mins
Cook:20 mins
Additional:5 mins
Servings:12

Ingredients

Cooking spray
12 large eggs
5 slices Fully Cooked Bacon
¼ teaspoon freshly ground black pepper
1 cup cherry tomatoes, quartered
½ cup fresh baby arugula leaves, chopped
½ cup shredded Cheddar cheese
½ teaspoon kosher salt
½ cup green onions, finely sliced
½ teaspoon hot sauce

Directions

Preheat oven to 350 degrees F and spray a 12-cup muffin tin lightly
with cooking spray.
    2
Crumble Smithfield® fully cooked bacon into small pieces and place
into a small bowl.
    3
Place eggs into a large mixing bowl. Whisk until combined. Add
bacon, tomatoes, arugula, cheese, green onions, salt, hot sauce, and
pepper. Whisk gently until Ingredients are combined.
    4

Use a 1/3 cup to pour egg mixture into prepared muffin cups. Bake for 25 minutes, or until eggs are set. Remove and let sit for 3 to 5 minutes before transferring to serving plates. Serve warm.

Nutrition

103 calories
protein 8.1g
carbohydrates 1.4g
fat 7.3g
cholesterol 193mg
sodium 217mg.

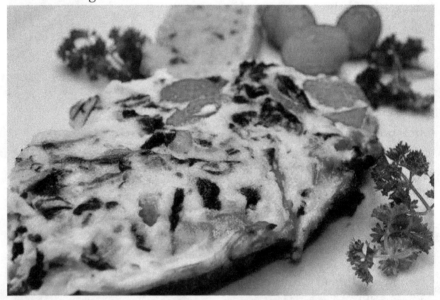

Cheddar and Spinach Muffins

Prep:20 mins
Cook:35 mins
Servings:12

Ingredients

1 ½ cups all-purpose flour
1 egg
2 teaspoons baking powder
½ teaspoon salt
6 tablespoons butter, melted
½ teaspoon baking soda
1 cup whole milk
1 cup shredded Cheddar cheese
1 cup frozen chopped spinach - thawed, drained and squeezed dry

Directions

Preheat oven to 350 degrees F.
Lightly grease 12 cup muffin cups.
2
Mix the flour, baking powder, baking soda, and salt together in a mixing bowl.
3
Stir the melted butter, egg, milk, spinach, and Cheddar cheese together in a large mixing bowl until evenly blended. Slowly stir in the flour mixture to form a batter. Spoon 2 tablespoons into each muffin cup.
4
Bake in preheated oven until a toothpick inserted into the center of a muffin comes out clean, about 30 minutes.

Nutrition

164 calories
protein 5.5g
carbohydrates 13.5g
fat 9.9g
cholesterol 42.3mg
sodium 349.3mg.

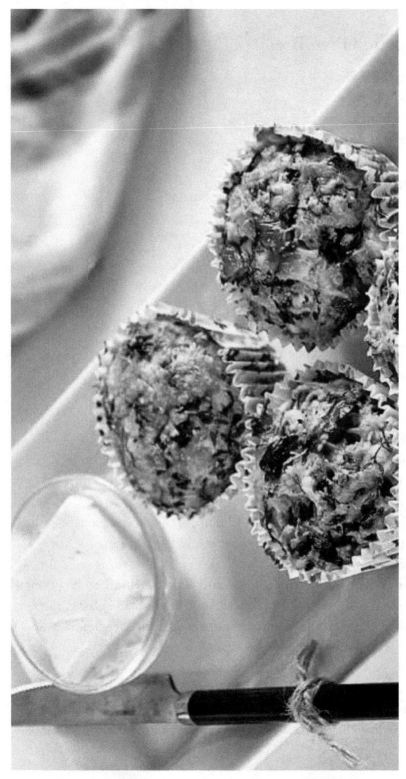

Rustic Olive Bread

Prep:20 mins
Cook:45 mins
Additional:2 hrs 15 mins
Servings:24

Ingredients

2 ½ cups warm water (110 degrees F)
2 tablespoons active dry yeast
1 tablespoon salt
7 ½ cups bread flour
1 teaspoon molasses
1 cup kalamata olives, pitted and chopped
2 tablespoons chopped fresh rosemary
2 tablespoons olive oil

Directions

Place water, yeast, and molasses in a mixing bowl; stir to mix. Let
stand for a few minutes until mixture is creamy and foamy.

2

Add olive oil and salt; mix. Add flour, about a cup at a time, until
dough is too stiff to stir. Add olives and fresh herbs.

3

Turn dough out onto a lightly floured board. Knead, adding flour as
needed to keep from being sticky, until smooth and elastic. Place in
well oiled bowl, and turn to coat the dough surface with oil. Allow to
rise until doubled in bulk, about an hour or so.

4

Punch the dough down, split into two pieces, and form into two round
loaves. Place on greased baking sheet . Spray with cold water and
sprinkle with sesame seeds if desired. Let loaves rise for 30 minutes.

5

Bake at 400 degrees F for 45 minutes.

Nutrition

186 calories
protein 5.7g;
carbohydrates 32.3g;
fat 3.6g;
sodium 383.9mg.

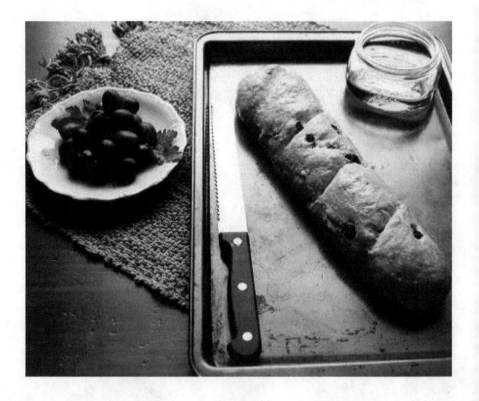

Pork with Arugula

Total:30 mins
Yield:4

Ingredients

2 tablespoons olive oil
1 1/2 pounds pork tenderloin, cut into 1-inch-thick medallions
Salt and freshly ground pepper
2 tablespoons balsamic vinegar
2 large garlic cloves, minced
1 pound arugula, stems discarded and leaves chopped
1 pound plum tomatoes, chopped
5 ounces thinly sliced prosciutto, finely chopped

Directions

In a very large skillet, heat the olive oil. Add the prosciutto and garlic and cook over moderate heat, stirring, until the garlic is golden, about 4 minutes. Transfer to a plate.

2

Season the pork medallions with salt and pepper, add them to the skillet and cook over moderately high heat until well browned on the outside and medium within, 4 minutes per side. Transfer the medallions to a plate and keep warm.

3

Add the balsamic vinegar to the skillet and cook until nearly evaporated, scraping up any browned bits from the bottom of the skillet. Add the arugula and toss until wilted, 2 minutes. Add the tomatoes and the prosciutto and garlic. Cook over high heat for 2 minutes, stirring occasionally; season with salt and pepper. Transfer the arugula to a platter, top with the pork and serve.

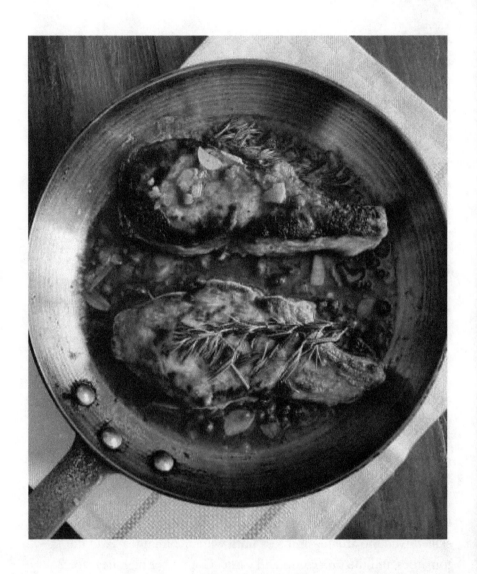

Mulligatawny

Prep:20 mins
Cook:1 hr
Servings:6

Ingredients

½ cup chopped onion
¼ cup butter
2 stalks celery, chopped
1 carrot, diced
1 ½ tablespoons all-purpose flour
4 cups chicken broth
½ apple, cored and chopped
¼ cup white rice
1 ½ teaspoons curry powder
1 skinless, boneless chicken breast half - cut into cubes
salt to taste
ground black pepper to taste
½ cup heavy cream, heated
1 pinch dried thyme

Directions

Saute onions, celery, carrot, and butter in a large soup pot. Add flour and curry, and cook 5 more minutes. Add chicken stock, mix well, and bring to a boil. Simmer about 1/2 hour.

2

Add apple, rice, chicken, salt, pepper, and thyme. Simmer 15-20 minutes, or until rice is done.

3

When serving, add hot cream.

Nutrition

223 calories; protein 6.9g; carbohydrates 13.5g; fat 15.8g; cholesterol 62.2mg; sodium 733.9mg.

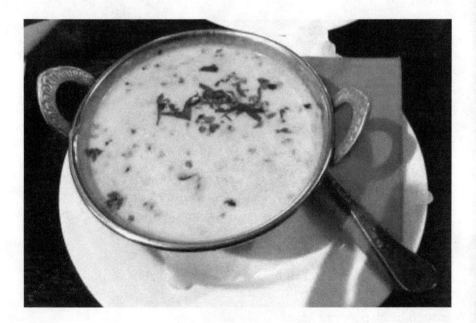

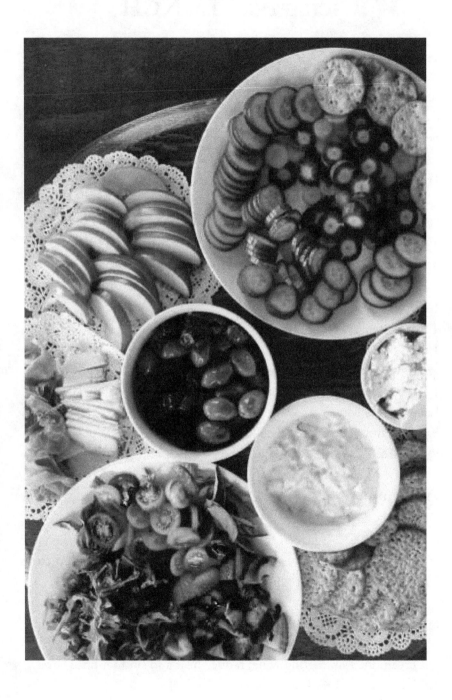

CHAPTER 4: LUNCH

Pasta with Chicken and Asparagus

Prep:20 mins
Cook:15 mins
Servings:8

Ingredients

⅓ cup corn oil
4 Roma tomatoes, chopped
4 skinless, boneless chicken breast halves, cubed
4 cloves garlic, minced
1 cup heavy whipping cream
4 Roma tomatoes, chopped
1 teaspoon salt
ground black pepper to taste
1 (16 ounce) package fresh linguini pasta
½ cup white wine
1 pound fresh asparagus, sliced
½ cup freshly grated Parmesan cheese

Directions

Heat corn oil in a skillet over medium heat. Cook and stir chicken and garlic until chicken is no longer pink in the center and juices run clear, 5 to 7 minutes. Transfer chicken to a plate.

2
Pour wine in the same skillet and simmer, about 2 minutes.

3
Stir cream into simmering wine; reduce heat and simmer until large bubbles appear, 3 to 4 minutes.

4

Cook and stir chicken, tomatoes, salt, and black pepper into cream mixture until all Ingredients are warmed, 2 minutes.

5

Bring a large pot of lightly salted water to a boil. Stir in pasta and asparagus; cook until pasta floats to the top, 3 minutes. Drain.

6

Toss pasta and asparagus together with chicken and cream sauce. Top with Parmesan cheese.

Nutrition

494 calories; protein 25.4g; carbohydrates 42g; fat 24g; cholesterol 125.6mg; sodium 431.1mg.

BEET SALAD

Prep:20 mins
Cook:45 mins
Servings:16

Ingredients

4 bunches fresh small beets, stems removed
2 tablespoons olive oil
2 tablespoons white wine vinegar
1 tablespoon honey
1 teaspoon dried thyme, crushed
½ cup vegetable oil
1 tablespoon lemon juice
salt and pepper to taste
2 medium heads Belgian endive
1 pound spring lettuce mix
1 cup crumbled feta cheese
2 tablespoons Dijon mustard

Directions

Preheat oven to 450 degrees F . Coat beets lightly with oil and roast
for approximately 45 minutes, or until tender. Allow to cool
thoroughly, then peel and dice.
  2
For the dressing, place lemon, vinegar, honey, mustard, and thyme in a
blender. While blender is running, gradually add 1/2 cup of oil. Season
to taste with salt and pepper. Place spring lettuce mix in a salad bowl,
pour desired amount of dressing over greens, and toss to coat.
  3

Rinse endive, tear off whole leaves, and pat dry. Arrange 3 leaves on each plate. Divide dressed salad greens among them, and top with diced beets and feta cheese.

Nutrition

166 calories; protein 4.2g; carbohydrates 14.9g; fat 10.8g; cholesterol 8.3mg; sodium 253.6mg.

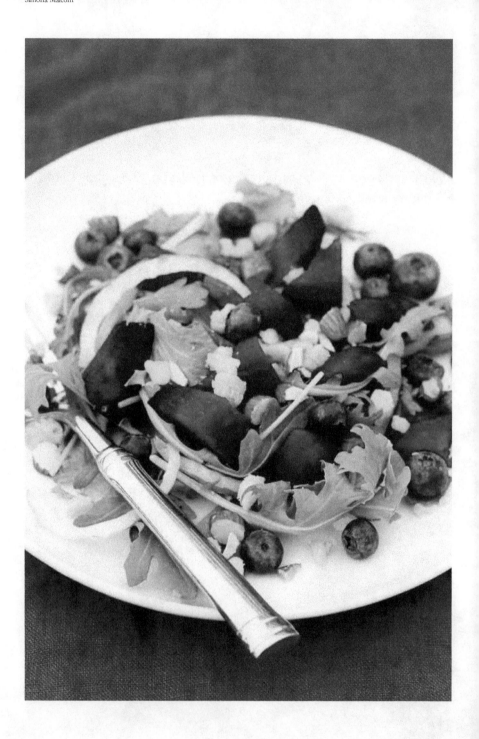

Orzo Salad

Prep:1 hr 10 mins
Cook:10 mins
Servings:6

Ingredients

1 ½ cups uncooked orzo pasta
½ teaspoon lemon pepper
1 tomato, seeded and chopped
1 cucumber, seeded and chopped
1 red onion, chopped
 (2 ounce) can black olives, drained
2 (6 ounce) cans marinated artichoke hearts
¼ cup chopped fresh parsley
1 tablespoon lemon juice
½ teaspoon dried oregano
1 cup crumbled feta cheese

Directions

Bring a large pot of lightly salted water to a boil. Add pasta and cook
for 8 to 10 minutes or until al dente; drain. Drain artichoke hearts,
reserving liquid.
    2
In large bowl combine pasta, artichoke hearts, tomato, cucumber,
onion, feta, olives, parsley, lemon juice, oregano and lemon pepper.
Toss and chill for 60 minutes in refrigerator.
    3
Just before serving, drizzle reserved artichoke marinade over salad.

Nutrition

:

326 calories; protein 13.1g; carbohydrates 48.7g; fat 10.2g; cholesterol 22.3mg; sodium 615.2mg.

HEALTHY BBQ SALAD

Prep:15 mins
Cook:12 mins
Additional:8 mins
Servings:8

Ingredients

2 skinless, boneless chicken breast halves
1 head red leaf lettuce, rinsed and torn
1 fresh tomato, chopped
1 bunch cilantro, chopped
½ cup barbeque sauce
1 (15.25 ounce) can whole kernel corn, drained
1 (15 ounce) can black beans, drained
1 (2.8 ounce) can French fried onions
1 head green leaf lettuce, rinsed and torn
½ cup Ranch dressing

Directions

Preheat the grill for high heat.
   2
Lightly oil the grill grate. Place chicken on the grill, and cook 6
minutes per side, or until juices run clear. Remove from heat, cool, and
slice.
   3
In a large bowl, mix the red leaf lettuce, green leaf lettuce, tomato,
cilantro, corn, and black beans. Top with the grilled chicken slices and
French fried onions.
   4
In a small bowl, mix the Ranch dressing and barbeque sauce. Serve on
the side as a dipping sauce, or toss with the salad to coat.

Nutrition

301 calories; protein 12.2g; carbohydrates 32.3g; fat 14.4g; cholesterol 20.8mg; sodium 805.4mg.

Mint Pesto Zucchini Noodles

Prep Time25 minutes
Total Time25 minutes
Servings4

Ingredients
1/4 cup sliced almonds, toasted
1 cup mint leaves
1/4 cup extra-virgin olive oil
1/4 cup fresh dill
1 clove garlic chopped
1/4 cup grated Parmesan cheese
2 tbsp lemon juice
3 medium zucchini
Salt and pepper to taste

Directions

For the almonds:
Heat oven to 350°F. Place slivered almonds in a single layer on a
baking sheet, and toast for 8 minutes, or until they have browned
slightly and just become fragrant. Remove the sheet from the oven and
immediately place almonds on a plate or in a bowl.
For the mint pesto:
Add mint leaves, dill, and garlic to the bowl of a food processor and
process until the herbs are finely broken up. Add olive oil, Parmesan,
lemon juice, and salt and pepper and process until creamy.
For the zucchini noodles:
Slice the very ends off of three zucchini and spiralize using the fine
spiralizer blade (or your blade of choice). Add the zucchini noodles to
a large mixing bowl and pour in the pesto sauce. Toss to combine.

Top with additional Parmesan, dill, mint, and/or toasted almonds for serving, along with your favorite protein if making this a full meal.

Nutrition

Calories: 169kcal | Carbohydrates: 6.5g | Protein: 4.5g | Fat: 15.4g | S aturated
Fat: 2.9g | Cholesterol: 4mg | Sodium: 150mg | Potassium: 452mg | Fiber: 2.2g | Sugar: 2.8g | Calcium: 70mg | Iron: 1.1mg

Caramelized Onions

Prep:10 mins
Cook:25 mins
Servings:4

Ingredients

6 slices bacon, chopped
2 tablespoons molasses
¼ teaspoon salt
¼ teaspoon pepper
2 sweet onions, cut into thin strips

Directions

Place bacon in a heavy skillet. Cook over medium-high heat until crisp. Remove bacon, reserving 1 tablespoon drippings in skillet. Crumble bacon, and set aside.
Cook onions in reserved drippings for 15 minutes, or until onion is soft and caramel colored. Stir in molasses, salt and pepper. Place in a serving dish, and sprinkle with crumbled bacon.

Nutrition

244 calories; protein 5.5g; carbohydrates 13g; fat 19g; cholesterol 28.6mg; sodium 501.2mg.

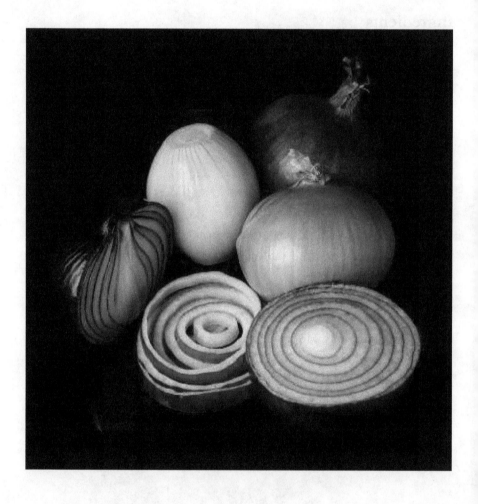

Snickers Caramel Apple Salad

Prep:10 mins
Additional:30 mins
Servings:12

Ingredients

1 (8 ounce) container frozen whipped topping, thawed
1 (8 ounce) can crushed pineapple
1 (3.4 ounce) package instant butterscotch pudding mix
1 cup skinless peanuts
2 cups chopped apples

Directions

Stir whipped topping, pineapple, and butterscotch pudding mix together in a bowl until smooth. Fold apples and peanuts into pudding mixture until salad is well mixed.
Refrigerate salad until completely chilled, at least 30 minutes.

Nutrition

181 calories; protein 3.2g; carbohydrates 20g; fat 10.8g; sodium 227.7mg.

Mince with Basil

0:30 Prep
0:15 Cook
6 Servings

INGREDIENTS

1 iceberg lettuce
2 tablespoons vegetable oil
500g lean beef mince
1 tablespoon white sugar
3 long red chillies, sliced
4 cloves garlic, finely chopped
2 tablespoons fish sauce
1 tablespoon oyster sauce
1/2 cup Massel chicken style liquid stock
1/3 cup basil leaves, shredded
3 green onions, thinly sliced
Select all ingredients

Directions

Remove core from lettuce. Cut in half lengthways and place into a large bowl of cold water. Allow to stand for 30 minutes. This loosens the leaves and enables easy peeling to form cups.

Heat oil in a large frypan over high heat. Add half the mince and cook, stirring continuously, until well-browned. Remove and repeat with remaining mince.

Return mince to pan and add chillies, garlic, fish sauce, sugar, oyster sauce, and stock. Stir until well-combined. Bring to the boil. Reduce the heat to medium-low and simmer. Add green onions and cook for 4 minutes.

Remove from heat and fold through basil. Spoon the chilli mince beef into the lettuce cups and serve immediately.

Vegetable Masala

Prep:10 mins
Cook:20 mins
Servings:4

Ingredients

2 potatoes, peeled and cubed
10 French-style green beans, chopped
1 quart cold water
½ cup frozen green peas, thawed
1 carrot, chopped
1 teaspoon salt
½ teaspoon ground turmeric
1 tablespoon vegetable oil
1 teaspoon ground cumin
1 onion, finely chopped
2 tomatoes - blanched, peeled and chopped
1 teaspoon mustard seed
1 teaspoon garam masala
½ teaspoon garlic powder
½ teaspoon chili powder
½ teaspoon ground ginger
1 sprig cilantro leaves, for garnish

Directions

Place potatoes, carrots and green beans in the cold water. Allow to soak while you prepare the rest of the vegetables; drain.
In a microwave safe dish place the potatoes, carrots, green beans, peas, salt and turmeric. Cook for 8 minutes.
Heat oil in a large skillet over medium heat. Cook mustard seeds and cumin; when seeds start to sputter and pop, add the onion and saute

until transparent. Stir in the tomatoes, garam masala, ginger, garlic and chili powder; saute 3 minutes. Add the cooked vegetables to the tomato mixture and saute 1 minute. Garnish with cilantro leaves.

Nutrition

168 calories; protein 4.2g; carbohydrates 29.8g; fat 4.3g; sodium 641.3mg.

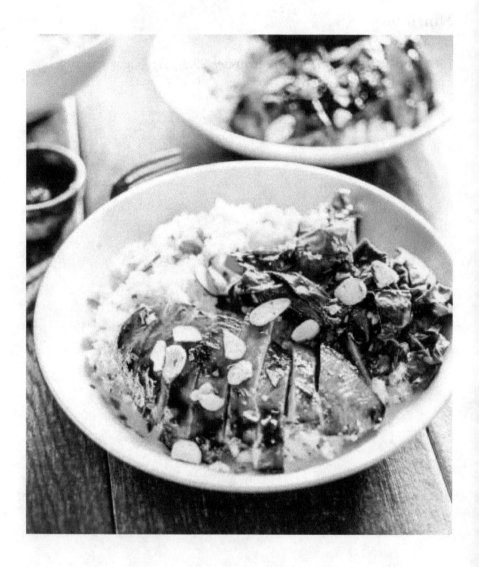

CHAPTER 5: DINNER

Beef Burritos

Prep:30 mins
Cook:20 mins
Servings:6

Ingredients

6 ounces sliced jalapeno peppers
1 tomato, diced
1 green bell pepper, diced
1 red bell pepper, diced
1 onion, diced
1 ½ tablespoons hot sauce
¼ teaspoon ground cayenne pepper
1 (4 ounce) can chopped green chile peppers
1 pound ground beef
1 (14 ounce) can refried beans
6 (10 inch) flour tortillas
1 (10 ounce) bag shredded lettuce
1 (1 ounce) package burrito seasoning
1 (8 ounce) package shredded sharp Cheddar cheese
1 (8 ounce) container sour cream

Directions

Mix jalapeno peppers, tomato, green chile peppers, green bell pepper, red bell pepper, onion, hot sauce, and cayenne pepper together in a large bowl.

Cook beef in a large skillet over medium-high heat, stirring to break up clumps, about 5 minutes. Drain excess grease. Add jalapeno pepper mixture and burrito seasoning; cook, covered, stirring occasionally, until flavors combine, about 10 minutes.

Pour refried beans into a saucepan over medium-low heat. Cook and stir until heated through, about 5 minutes.

Warm each tortilla in the microwave until soft, 15 to 20 seconds. Spread a layer of refried beans on top. Divide beef mixture among tortillas. Top with lettuce, sour cream, and Cheddar cheese. Fold in opposing edges of each tortilla and roll up into a burrito.

Nutrition

723 calories; protein 34g; carbohydrates 59.9g; fat 38.9g; cholesterol 107.5mg; sodium 2042.5mg.

White Fish Soup

PREP TIME10 mins
COOK TIME20 mins
SERVINGS4 servings

Ingredients

6 tablespoons extra virgin olive oil
1 medium onion, chopped (about 1 1/2 cups)
3 large garlic cloves, minced
1/8 teaspoon freshly ground black pepper
2/3 cup fresh parsley, chopped
1 1/2 cups of fresh chopped tomato (about 1 medium sized tomato)
OR 1 14-ounce can of whole or crushed tomatoes with their juices
1/2 cup dry white wine (like Sauvignon blanc)
1 1/2 pound fish fillets (use a firm white fish such as halibut, cod, red
snapper, or sea bass), cut into 2-inch pieces
Pinch of dry oregano
8 oz of clam juice
Pinch of dry thyme
1/8 teaspoon Tabasco sauce
1 teaspoon of salt

Directions

Sauté aromatics:
Heat olive oil in a large thick-bottomed pot over medium-high heat.
Add onion and sauté 4 minutes, add the garlic and cook a minute
more. Add parsley and stir 2 minutes. Add tomato and tomato paste,
and gently cook for 10 minutes or so.
Finish soup:
Add clam juice, dry white wine, and fish. Bring to a simmer and
simmer until the fish is cooked through and easily flakes apart, about 3

to 5 minutes. Add seasoning —salt, pepper, oregano, thyme, Tabasco. Add more salt and pepper to taste. Ladle into bowls and serve. Great served with crusty bread for dipping in the fish stew broth.

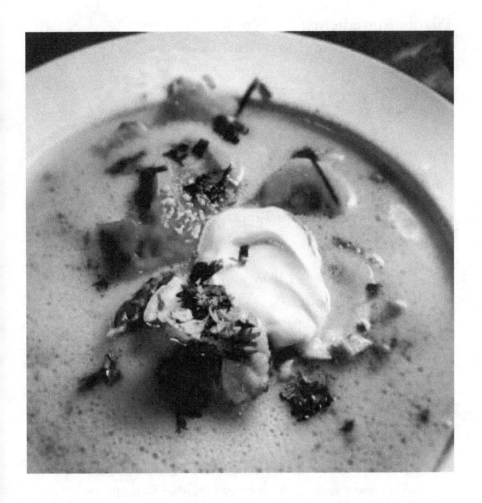

Tilapia Casserole

Prep 10 mins
Cook: 40 mins
Servings: 7

Tilapia Ingredients:

2 lbs (about 6-10 count) Tilapia fillets, thawed
Olive Oil to saute
1 Tbsp mayo
1 Tbsp ketchup

Marinade Ingredients:

2 large eggs
1 cup buttermilk
1/2 tsp Salt and 1/8 teaspoon Pepper
2 Tbsp soy sauce
Vegetable Ingredients:
2 medium bell peppers (red, orange, or yellow)
1 medium onion
2 medium/large carrots, julienned or grated

Directions:

Whisk together marinade ingredients. Combine with tilapia in a large
ziploc bag or bowl and marinate in the fridge at least 1 1/2 hours.
Slice onions into thin half circles, slice bell pepper into thin strips
and julienne or grate carrots. In a large skillet over medium/high, heat
2-3 Tbsp oil and saute onions for 3 minutes or until softened. Add
sliced bell peppers and carrots and saute another 5 min or until
softened. Remove from pan and set veggies aside.
Once fish is done marinating, drain and discard marinade. In the same
empty skillet over medium/high, add 2-3 Tbsp oil and saute fish lightly
on the skillet just until golden on the outside (2 min per side) – it's ok
if it's not cooked through completely at this point.

Layer the casserole dish with 1/2 of the vegetables on the bottom. Place fish over the vegetables. Stir together 1 Tbsp ketchup and 1 Tbsp mayo and brush this mixture evenly over the top of the fish. Cover fish with remaining veggies. Sprinkle the top with salt and pepper

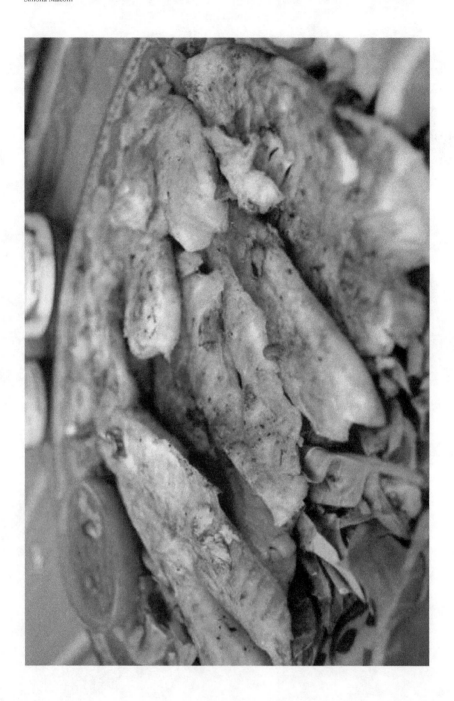

Cumin Beef

Cook: 15 mins
Prep: 5 mins
Servings: 2

Ingredients

700 g rump Beef
4 teaspoon finely chopped ginger
4 fresh red chilli, seeded, finely chopped
4 spring onions only the green parts, in very fine rings
4-8 teaspoon dried chilli flakes
4 teaspoon ground cumin
2 tablespoons finely chopped garlic
salt
500 ml Plenty of oil for frying
Marinade
2 tablespoons Shaoxing wine
1 sachet of baking powder
2 teaspoon light soy sauce
1 teaspoon salt
2 teaspoon dark soy sauce
2 tablespoons water
2 tablespoons potato starch

DIRECTIONS

Cut meat against the grain into thin slices about 4 cm x 3 cm and then marinate.

The oil in a wok heat up to around 140 ° C. pour in meat in two stages, and stir thoroughly. Once the pieces separate from each other, remove and allow to drain well on the large slotted spoon.

Drain Oil up to 4 tbsp. Then add in strong flame ginger, garlic, fresh chilies, possibly pepper flakes and cumin and stir fry briefly. give meat back into the wok and mix well, season with salt.

When all the ingredients sizzle nice and smell good, the F-onion rings fold briefly take wok from the heat, stir in sesame oil and serve.

Chow Mein

Prep:20 mins
Cook:15 mins
Additional:20 mins
Servings:4

Ingredients

2 teaspoons soy sauce
¼ teaspoon sesame oil
½ pound skinless, boneless chicken breast halves, cut into strips
¾ cup chicken broth
1 teaspoon cornstarch
2 tablespoons oyster sauce
1 carrot, cut into thin strips
½ pound chow mein noodles
1 teaspoon minced garlic
2 heads bok choy, chopped
½ zucchini, diced
¾ teaspoon white sugar
1 tablespoon vegetable oil
10 sugar snap peas
2 tablespoons chopped green onion

Directions

Whisk soy sauce, corn starch, and sesame oil together in a large bowl until smooth; add chicken strips and toss to coat. Cover and refrigerate for at least 20 minutes.

Combine chicken broth, oyster sauce, and sugar in a small bowl and set aside.

Bring a large pot of water to a boil. Add noodles and cook over medium heat until cooked through but still firm to the bite, 4 to 6 minutes. Drain and rinse with cold water.

Heat vegetable oil in a large skillet. Cook and garlic in hot oil for 30 seconds; add marinated chicken. Cook and stir until browned and no longer pink in the center, 5 to 6 minutes. Remove chicken mixture to a plate. Cook and stir bok choy, zucchini, snap peas, and carrot in the hot skillet until softened, about 2 minutes. Return noodles and chicken mixture to the skillet. Pour broth mixture into noodle mixture; cook and stir until warmed through, about 2 minutes. Serve garnished with green onions.

Nutrition

527 calories; protein 29.4g; carbohydrates 61.7g; fat 17.9g; cholesterol 30.2mg; sodium 991.7mg.

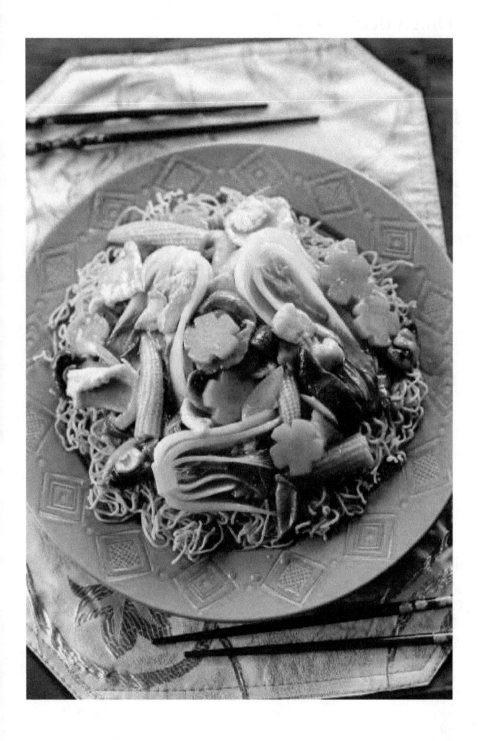

Onion Beef Gravy

Prep:5 mins
Cook:36 mins
Servings:8

Ingredients

cooking spray
1 (1 ounce) package dry onion soup mix
1 teaspoon beef base (such as Better Than Bouillon®)
1 teaspoon minced garlic
3 cups water
3 tablespoons all-purpose flour
¼ cup milk
ground black pepper to taste

Directions

Spray a saucepan with cooking spray. Add garlic and cook over
medium heat just until fragrant, about 1 minute. Add water, onion
soup mix, and beef base; bring to a boil. Cover the pan and simmer
until onions are tender, about 20 minutes.
Combine milk and flour in a jar with a lid; shake until combined and
whisk into the saucepan. Bring gravy back to a boil and cook until
thickened, about 10 minutes. Season with black pepper.

Nutrition

26 calories; protein 0.9g; carbohydrates 5.1g; fat 0.3g; cholesterol
0.6mg; sodium 370.4mg

Salad with Brie and Apple

Prep:10 mins
Total:10 mins
Servings:4

Ingredients

½ cup balsamic vinaigrette
½ cup sliced Brie cheese
3 cups spring mix salad greens
2 red apples, cored and thinly sliced
⅓ cup toasted walnut pieces

Directions

Toss the apple slices with the vinaigrette in a bowl until evenly coated; add the greens and toss again; top with the Brie and walnuts just before serving.

Nutrition
:
258 calories; protein 6.1g; carbohydrates 15.2g; fat 20.7g; cholesterol 18mg; sodium 474.6mg.

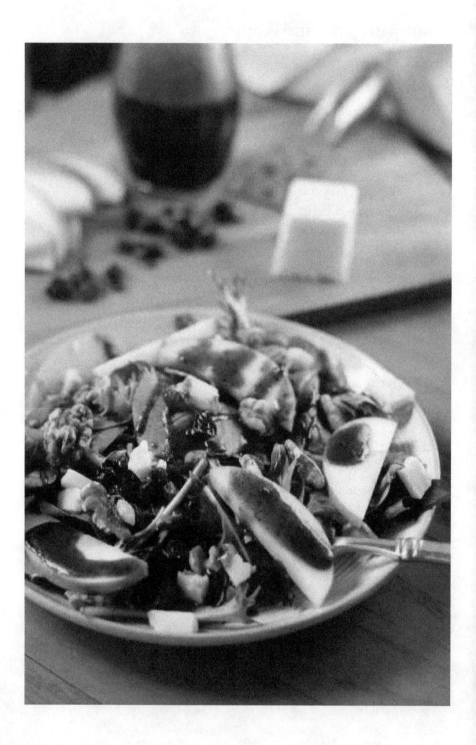

Alfredo Sauce Pasta

Prep:5 mins
Cook:5 mins
Servings:4

Ingredients

1 (8 ounce) package cream cheese
2 teaspoons garlic powder
2 cups milk
6 ounces grated Parmesan cheese
½ cup butter
⅛ teaspoon ground black pepper

Directions

Melt butter in a medium, non-stick saucepan over medium heat. Add cream cheese and garlic powder, stirring with wire whisk until smooth. Add milk, a little at a time, whisking to smooth out lumps. Stir in Parmesan and pepper. Remove from heat when sauce reaches desired consistency. Sauce will thicken rapidly, thin with milk if cooked too long. Toss with hot pasta to serve.

Nutrition

648 calories; protein 25.1g; carbohydrates 10g; fat 57.1g; cholesterol 169.8mg; sodium 1029.8mg.

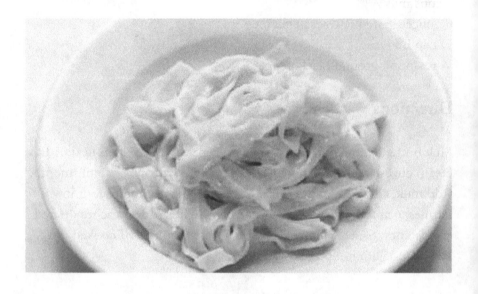

Crab Stew

Serves 6

Ingredients

12 large live blue crabs
½ cup all-purpose flour
1¼ cups chopped onion
¼ cup vegetable oil
¼ cup chopped green bell pepper
¾ cup chopped celery
2 bay leaves
¼ cup chopped red bell pepper
1 teaspoon salt
6 cups seafood stock
1 pound lump crabmeat, picked free of shells
½ teaspoon cayenne pepper
1½ pounds large fresh shrimp, peeled and deveined
2 tablespoons finely chopped fresh parsley

Directions

Scald crabs with hot water to stun. Remove the back shell (top shell) from each crab, and clean out gills, lungs, and center of each. Crack crabs in half, and remove claws. Reserve claws for stock.
In a large heavy stockpot, combine oil and flour, and heat over medium heat. Stirring slowly, make a dark-brown roux, 15 to 20 minutes. Add onion, bell peppers, and celery. Cook, stirring frequently, until vegetables are soft, about 5 minutes. Add bay leaves, salt, cayenne, and seafood stock. Stir to combine. Bring mixture to a boil over high heat; reduce heat to medium-low, add crabs, and simmer 20 minutes. Add crabmeat and shrimp, and cook 10 minutes. Remove from heat, and add parsley. Serve hot.

Lime Lobsters

Serves: 4 People
Prep time: 15m
Cook Time: 10m

Ingredients

4 Lobster tails (6-7 oz.)
1/2 Teaspoon Paprika
2 Tablespoons Lime Juice
1 Tablespoon Olive Oil
2 Tablespoons Butter

Directions

Rinse lobster tails: pat dry with paper towels. Use kitchen sheers to cut through hard top shell of lobster tail, cutting through meat, but not through the lower shell. Spread meat open in shell. Preheat broiler.
In a small bowl whisk together butter, like juice, olive oil and paprika. Place lobster tails, meat size up, on the broiler pan rack. Set aside 3 tablespoons of butter mixture; keep warm. Brush lobster meat with remaining butter mixture.
Broil 4 to 5 inches from heat for 6 minutes or until opaque in center. Be careful NOT to overcook. Drizzle with reserved butter mixture.

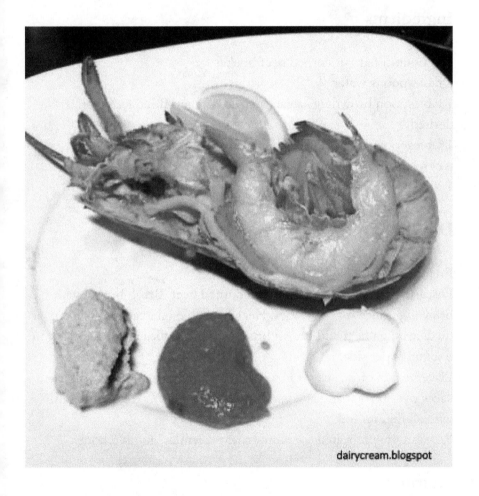

dairycream.blogspot

Beef Brisket

Prep:15 mins
Cook:6 hrs 15 mins
Servings:6

Ingredients

1 (5 pound) flat-cut corned beef brisket
2 tablespoons water
1 tablespoon browning sauce (such as Kitchen Bouquet®), or as
desired
1 tablespoon vegetable oil
6 cloves garlic, sliced
1 onion, sliced

Directions

Preheat oven to 275 degrees F .
Discard any flavoring packet from corned beef. Brush brisket with
browning sauce on both sides. Heat vegetable oil in a large skillet over
medium-high heat and brown brisket on both sides in the hot oil, 6 to
8 minutes per side.
Place brisket on a rack set in a roasting pan. Scatter onion and garlic
slices over brisket and add water to roasting pan. Cover pan tightly
with aluminum foil.
Roast in the preheated oven until meat is tender, about 6 hours.

Nutrition

:
455 calories; protein 30.6g; carbohydrates 5.4g; fat 33.7g; cholesterol
162mg; sodium 1877.4mg.

Yucatan Soup

Cook Time2 hrs 30 mins
Total Time2 hrs 30 mins

Ingredients

For the Tortillas
lard (for frying)
1 package corn tortillas (sliced into strips)
For the Soup
1 white onion thinly sliced
3 limes
1 cup long-grain white rice
1 whole chicken (about 3 pounds)
To Serve
Jalapeños
Cotija cheese
limes
avocados

Directions

Line a plate with a paper towel or a cotton kitchen towel.
Set a cast-iron skillet over medium heat. Spoon enough lard into the skillet so that when it melts, it reaches about 1/2 inch up the side of the skillet, about 11/2 cups.
Once the fat melts completely and begins to shimmer in the skillet, test the oil by dropping a tortilla strip into the hot fat. If the tortilla sizzles immediately in the pan, crisping and turning a golden brown within about 30 seconds, the oil is ready. Working in batches, and taking care not to crowd the pan, fry the tortilla strips until crisp and golden brown. Using a slotted spoon, transfer the tortilla strips to the lined plate, and allow them to cool. Turn off the heat.

Place the whole chicken in a large stock pot. Pour enough water into the pot to cover the chicken by 2 inches. Bring the pot to a boil over medium-high heat, then immediately reduce the heat to medium-low and simmer, covered, for 2 hours, or until the chicken is cooked through and the meat shreds easily with a fork. Turn off the heat. Carefully remove the chicken from the pot, setting it on a platter to allow it to cool until it's comfortable enough to handle. Remove and discard the skin, pull the meat from the bone, and shred it with a fork. Strain the broth in the pot through a fine-mesh sieve into a pitcher or jar, discarding the solids. Wipe out the pot to remove any stray debris, and then return the strained broth and reserved chicken meat to the pot. Stir in the onion and rice and then bring to a simmer over medium heat. While the soup warms, juice one of the limes and then stir the juice into the soup pot. Continue cooking until the onion is soft and translucent and the chicken is warmed. While soup is cooking, finely chop the remaining 2 limes, peel and all.

Ladle into soup bowls and serve with the chopped lime, sliced jalapeño, crumbled Cotija cheese, sliced avocado, and tortilla strips.

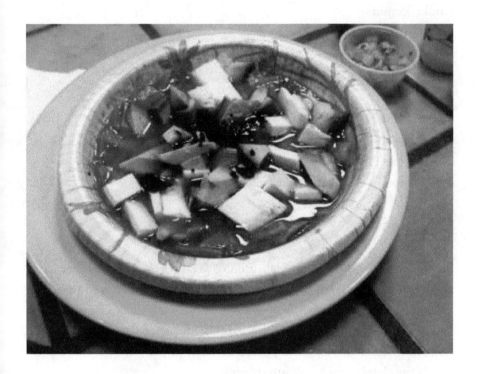

CHAPTER 6: SNACKS E SIDES RECIPES

Cinnamon Chips

Prep:5 mins
Cook: 35 mins
Servings: 24

Ingredients

⅓ cup white sugar
1 tablespoon light corn syrup
2 teaspoons ground cinnamon
1 tablespoon vegetable shortening

Directions

Stir sugar, ground cinnamon, shortening, and corn syrup together in a small bowl until dough comes together. Place dough between two layers of parchment paper; roll to 1/8- to 1/4-inch thick. Transfer to a baking sheet; remove top piece of parchment paper.
Bake in preheated oven until golden and bubbly, about 35 minutes. Cool completely and break into pieces.

Nutrition

18 calories; carbohydrates 3.6g; fat 0.5g; sodium 0.5mg.

Peas Hummus

Total Time: 5 minutes
Servings: 10

Ingredients

400 g (15 oz) can of chickpeas - not yet drained (garbanzo beans)
Pinch of salt and pepper
150 g (1 cup) fresh or frozen peas
2 tsp lemon juice
1 clove of garlic minced
2 tbsp tahini

Directions

Drain the chickpeas over a bowl to collect the liquid (aquafaba), then add the chickpeas to a blender or food processor.
Run the frozen peas under hot water to thaw, then also add them to the blender, along with the tahini, lemon juice, garlic salt and pepper as well as 4 tbsp of the aquafaba.
Blend for a few minutes until thick and creamy. You may need to scrape the sides down periodically. Add a little more aquafaba if necessary to get it a thick and creamy consistency.

Nutrition

Calories: 63kcal Carbohydrates: 8g Protein: 3g Fat: 2g Sodium: 3mg Po
tassium: 108mg Fiber: 2g Sugar: 1g Vitamin A: 120IU Vitamin
C: 6.8mg Calcium: 18mg Iron: 0.9mg

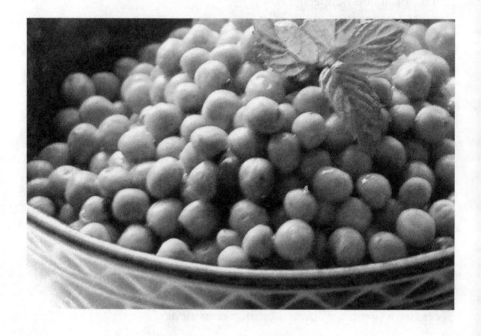

Mozzarella Cheese Cookies

Prep: 15 mins

Cook: 20 Mins

Servings: 4

INGREDIENTS

- 175g salted butter
- 175g Mozzarella cheese - grated
- 2 egg yolks
- 250g plain flour

DIRECTIONS

Add flour in a mixing bowl.

Remove butter from refrigerator and cut into small cubes.

Rub in the butter with your fingertips until the mixture resembles bread crumbs.

Add egg yolks and grated cheese. Mix with hands until a dough is formed.

Roll out the dough until it's about 5mm in thickness. Cut out the cookies with a cookie cutter.

Place about 2cm apart on a lined baking tray. Brush with egg wash.

Bake in preheated oven at 200 for 18-20 minutes, or till golden in color.

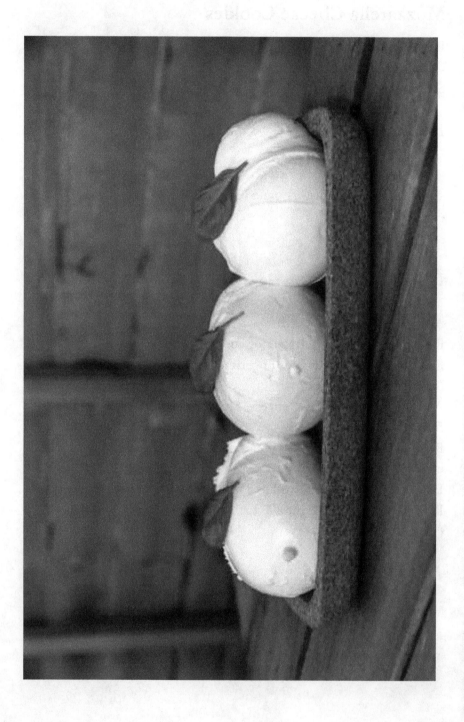

Dijon Mustard Vinaigrette

Total Time: 5 minutes
Makes: about 1 cup

Ingredients

1/4 cup white wine vinegar (or lemon juice)
2 tablespoons Dijon mustard
1/2 cup olive oil
1 garlic clove, minced
1/4 teaspoon black pepper
1/2 teaspoon coarse salt

Directions

Combine ingredients in a bowl.
Whisk until smooth and everything has emulsified.
Adjust seasoning with salt & pepper, to taste.

Nutrition

Serving Size: 2 tablespoons
Calories: 113
Sugar: 0.1g
Sodium: 165g
Fat: 12.8g
Saturated Fat: 1.8g
Carbohydrates: 0.5g
Fiber: 0.2g
Protein: 0.2g
Cholesterol: 0

Green Tomatillo Salsa

PREP TIME10 mins
COOK TIME15 mins
YIELDS3 cups

Ingredients

1 1/2 lb tomatillos
2 cloves garlic
1/2 cup cilantro leaves
1/2 cup chopped white onion
2 Jalapeño peppers OR 2 serrano peppers, stemmed, seeded and chopped
1 Tbsp fresh lime juice
Salt to taste

Directions

Remove papery husks from tomatillos and rinse well
3 ways to cook the tomatillos
2a Oven Roasting Method
Cut the tomatillos in half and place cut side down on a foil-lined baking sheet. Add a few garlic cloves in their skin (if using) Place under a broiler for about 6-8 minutes to lightly blacken the skins of the tomatillos.
2b Pan Roasting Method
Coat the bottom of a skillet with a little vegetable oil. Heat on high heat. Place the tomatillos in the pan and sear on one side, then flip over and brown on the other side. Remove from heat.
2c Boiling Method
Place tomatillos in a saucepan, cover with water. Bring to a boil and simmer for 5 minutes. Remove tomatillos with a slotted spoon.
Pulse in blender

Place the cooked tomatillos, lime juice, onions, garlic (if using), cilantro, chili peppers in a blender or food processor and pulse until all ingredients are finely chopped and mixed.

Season to taste with salt.

Cool in refrigerator.

Serve with chips or as a salsa accompaniment to Mexican dishes.

Rutabaga Latkes

Prep Time10 mins
Cook Time20 mins
Servings: 10 Latkes

Ingredients

1 lb. peeled, grated rutabaga (approx. 3 cups)
1 egg, lightly beaten
1 Tbsp. coconut flour
1 scallion, minced
3-4 Tbsp. raw, shelled hemp seeds
1 tsp. salt
A few gratings of fresh nutmeg
Pepper to taste
Olive oil for frying

Directions

In a large bowl, add grated rutabaga, minced scallion, beaten egg, coconut flour, hemp seeds, salt, pepper and nutmeg. Mix well.
In a large skillet, heat a good tablespoon of olive oil between medium low and medium heat. Working in batches of 3 latkes, spoon about 2 tablespoons of mixture per latke into skillet, spreading into 3 to 4 inch rounds and frying until the edges begin to brown. Flip and fry until other side is golden brown. Repeat with remaining latke mixture, adding another good tablespoon of olive oil to the skillet for each batch.
When latkes are done frying, place in warm oven on wire racks on a rimmed baking sheet. This keeps latkes crispy until ready to serve.

CHAPTER 7: DESSERTS

Chocolate Cake

Servings:12

Ingredients

1 (18.25 ounce) package devil's food cake mix
½ cup warm water
1 (5.9 ounce) package instant chocolate pudding mix
1 cup vegetable oil
4 eggs
1 cup sour cream
2 cups semisweet chocolate chips

Directions

Preheat oven to 350 degrees F.
In a large bowl, mix together the cake and pudding mixes, sour cream, oil, beaten eggs and water. Stir in the chocolate chips and pour batter into a well greased 12 cup bundt pan.
Bake for 50 to 55 minutes, or until top is springy to the touch and a wooden toothpick inserted comes out clean. Cool cake thoroughly in pan at least an hour and a half before inverting onto a plate If desired, dust the cake with powdered sugar.

Nutrition

600 calories; protein 7.6g; carbohydrates 60.9g; fat 38.6g; cholesterol 78.9mg; sodium 550.4mg.

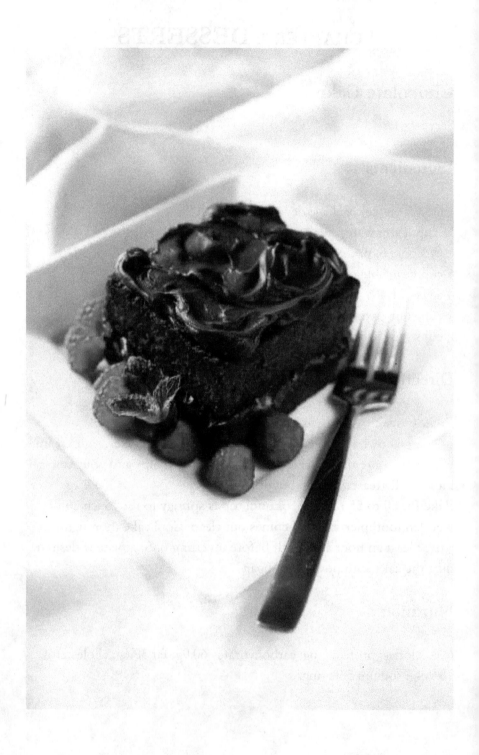

Crab Cakes

Prep:25 mins
Cook:20 mins
Servings:6

Ingredients

⅓ cup dry bread crumbs
¼ red bell pepper, seeded and diced
2 green onions, thinly sliced
¼ green bell pepper, seeded and diced
½ teaspoon hot pepper sauce
1 egg white
2 tablespoons mayonnaise
1 cup canola oil for frying
4 sprigs fresh parsley, chopped
1 tablespoon fresh lemon juice
2 teaspoons Dijon mustard
¼ teaspoon Old Bay TM seasoning
¼ teaspoon dry mustard
½ teaspoon Worcestershire sauce
3 (6 ounce) cans crabmeat, drained and flaked
½ cup dry bread crumbs
¼ teaspoon onion powder

Directions

In a bowl, toss together the 1/3 cup bread crumbs, green bell pepper, red bell pepper, green onions, and parsley. Mix in the egg white, mayonnaise, lemon juice, Worcestershire sauce, and Dijon mustard. Season with Old Bay seasoning, dry mustard, and onion powder. Fold crabmeat into the mixture. Form into 6 large cakes. Coat in the remaining 1/2 cup bread crumbs.

Heat the oil in a large, heavy skillet. Fry the cakes 5 minutes on each side, or until evenly brown. Drain on paper towels.

Nutrition

225 calories; protein 20.7g; carbohydrates 13.8g; fat 9.4g; cholesterol 76.5mg; sodium 508mg

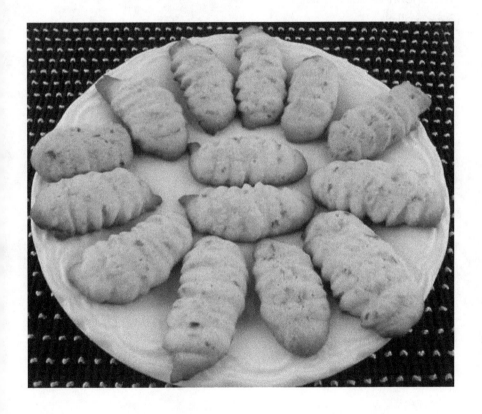

Spritz Cookies

Servings:24

Ingredients

1 cup butter, softened
1 teaspoon vanilla extract
3 egg yolks
⅔ cup white sugar
2 ½ cups all-purpose flour

Directions

Mix the butter or margarine, sugar, egg yolks and vanilla. Add the flour and mix by hand.
Spoon into cookie press and press onto ungreased cookie sheets.
Sprinkle with colored sugars.
Bake in preheated 400 degrees F oven for 8-10 minutes.

Nutrition

144 calories; protein 1.8g; carbohydrates 15.6g; fat 8.4g; cholesterol 45.9mg; sodium 55.8mg.

Blackberry Cobbler

Prep:20 mins
Cook:25 mins
Servings:8

Ingredients

1 cup all-purpose flour
1 ½ cups white sugar, divided
½ teaspoon salt
6 tablespoons cold butter
1 teaspoon baking powder
2 tablespoons cornstarch
¼ cup cold water
¼ cup boiling water
4 cups fresh blackberries, rinsed and drained
1 tablespoon lemon juice

Directions

Preheat oven to 400 degrees F . Line a baking sheet with aluminum foil.
In a large bowl, mix the flour, 1/2 cup sugar, baking powder, and salt. Cut in butter until the mixture resembles coarse crumbs. Stir in 1/4 cup boiling water just until mixture is evenly moist.
In a separate bowl, dissolve the cornstarch in cold water. Mix in remaining 1 cup sugar, lemon juice, and blackberries. Transfer to a cast iron skillet, and bring to a boil, stirring frequently. Drop dough into the skillet by spoonfuls. Place skillet on the foil lined baking sheet. Bake 25 minutes in the preheated oven, until dough is golden brown.

Nutrition

318 calories; protein 2.7g; carbohydrates 58.4g; fat 9.1g; cholesterol 22.9mg; sodium 253.3mg.

Chocolate Sorbet

Prep:5 mins
Cook:10 mins
Additional:3 hrs 20 mins
Servings:4

Ingredients

1 cup white sugar
⅛ teaspoon sea salt
2 cups water
2 tablespoons brewed espresso or strong coffee
½ teaspoon almond extract
⅔ cup unsweetened cocoa powder

Directions

Mix sugar, cocoa powder, and sea salt in a large saucepan. Stir in water, espresso, and almond extract. Bring to a boil over medium heat. Once the sugar has dissolved and mixture is smooth, remove from heat and stir in the coffee liqueur. Transfer mixture to a bowl, cover, and chill completely in the refrigerator or using an ice bath.
Pour mixture into an ice cream maker and churn until slightly thickened according to manufacturer's Directions, about 20 minutes. Transfer mixture to an airtight container and freeze until firm enough to scoop, 3 to 4 hours or overnight.

Nutrition

255 calories; protein 2.8g; carbohydrates 60.6g; fat 2g; sodium 63.3mg.

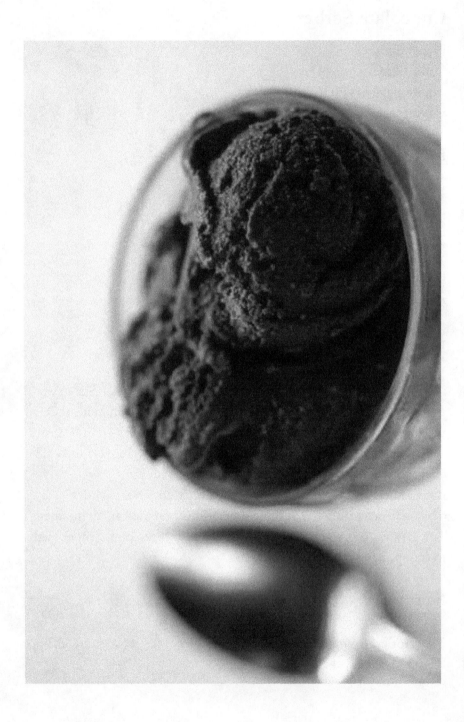

Banana Muffins

Prep:15 mins

Cook:30 mins

Servings:12

Ingredients

3 cups all-purpose flour

½ cup brown sugar

2 teaspoons ground cinnamon

1 cup white sugar

1 teaspoon baking soda

1 teaspoon ground nutmeg

1 teaspoon salt

2 teaspoons baking powder

2 cups mashed ripe bananas

1 cup coconut milk

1 cup canola oil

Directions

Preheat oven to 350 degrees F. Grease 12 muffin cups or line with paper liners.

Mix flour, white sugar, brown sugar, cinnamon, baking powder, baking soda, nutmeg, and salt together in a large bowl. Stir bananas, canola oil, and coconut milk together in a separate bowl; mix banana mixture into flour mixture until just combined. Fill muffin cups with batter. Bake in the preheated oven until a tooth pick inserted in the center of a muffin comes out clean, 30 to 35 minutes.

Nutrition

451 calories; protein 4.1g; carbohydrates 59.2g; fat 23.2g; sodium 386mg.

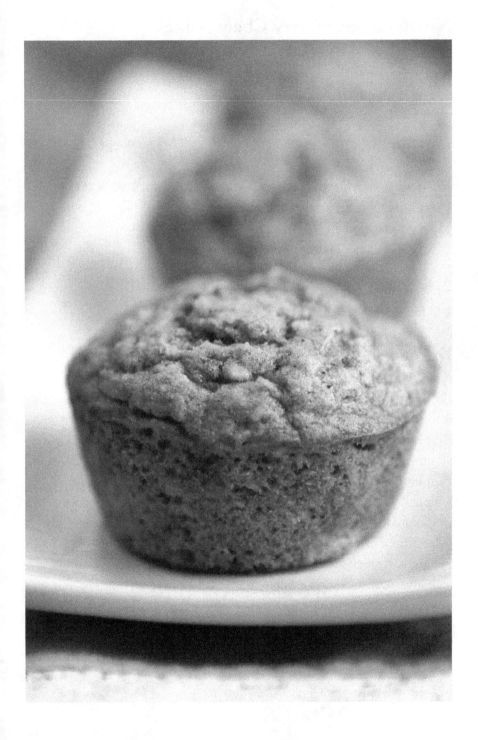

No-Bake Strawberry Cheesecake

Prep:30 mins
Additional:3 hrs 30 mins
Servings:10

Ingredients

1 (3 ounce) package strawberry-flavored gelatin (such as Jell-O®)
1 cup boiling water
1 cup white sugar
1 (5 ounce) can cold evaporated milk
1 teaspoon vanilla extract
1 (8 ounce) package cream cheese, softened
1 (9 inch) prepared graham cracker crust

Directions

Dissolve strawberry gelatin in boiling water in a bowl; cool in refrigerator until thick, but not set, about 20 minutes.
Beat cream cheese, sugar, and vanilla extract together in a bowl until smooth.
Beat evaporated milk in a separate bowl with an electric mixer until whipped and thick. Gradually pour strawberry gelatin mixture into evaporated milk, beating constantly. Fold cream cheese mixture into gelatin-milk mixture to form cheesecake filling.
Set graham cracker crust on a baking sheet or plate to maintain stability. Pour cheesecake filling into crust. Refrigerate until cake is set, at least 3 1/2 hours.

Nutrition

324 calories; protein 4.4g; carbohydrates 44.9g; fat 14.8g; cholesterol 28.7mg; sodium 252.7mg.

Cocoa Fat Bombs

Prep:20 mins
Cook:12 mins
Additional:4 hrs 28 mins
Servings:72

Ingredients

1/2 cup nut butter of choice or coconut butter
1/4 cup cocoa or cacao powder
1/4 cup melted coconut oil
stevia to taste, or 1 tbsp liquid sweetener of choice
optional, I like to add 1/8 tsp salt

Directions

Stir all ingredients together until smooth. If too dry (depending on nut butter used), add additional coconut oil if needed. Pour into a small container, ice cube trays, candy molds, or this silicone mini cupcake tin. Freeze to set. Because coconut oil softens when warm, it's best to store these in the freezer.

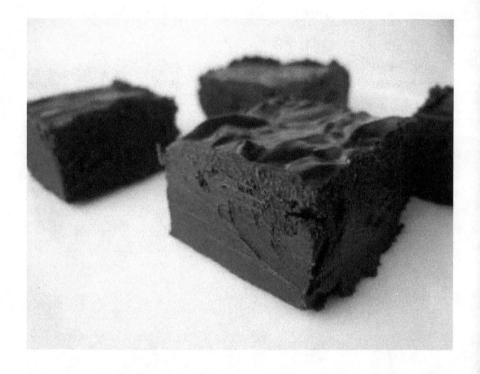

CHAPTER 8: SMOOTHIES AND DRINKS

Almonds and Zucchini Smoothie

Prep Time: 5 mins
Total Time: 5 mins

Ingredients

12 oz. unsweetened almond milk
1–2 scoop vanilla protein powder
1/2 cup frozen blueberries
1 TBS roasted almond butter
1 TBS ground chia seed
1 cup steamed and frozen green zucchini (or sub frozen caulilflower)

Directions

Ensure that you have steamed and frozen zucchini on hand or make it at least 8 hours in advance before starting recipe
Add all ingredients to high speed blender and process until smooth and creamy. Add more almond milk to reach thinner consistency and a little more blueberries or zucchini for thicker consistency. Pour into a large mason jar and enjoy topped with fresh blueberries, almond butter, and ground chia seeds.

Herbal Tea

Prep:5 mins
Cook:2 mins
Servings:4

Ingredients

1 quart water, or as needed
1 teaspoon ground cumin
1 teaspoon grated fresh ginger
1 tablespoon honey
1 teaspoon lime juice
3 leaves fresh mint
1 teaspoon grated lime zest

Directions

Bring water to a boil in a pot; stir in honey, cumin, ginger, lime zest, lime juice, and mint. Cook and stir until flavors are infused, about 2 minutes.

Nutrition

19 calories; protein 0.1g; carbohydrates 4.8g; fat 0.1g; sodium 8.3mg.

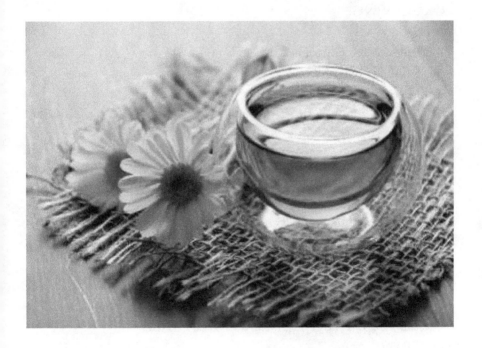

Honey Cinnamon Latte

INGREDIENTS

FOR THE SIMPLE SYRUP:
¾ cup honey
1 ½ teaspoons vanilla extract
3 cinnamon sticks
¾ cup water
FOR SERVING:
ice cubes
cold brew coffee concentrate
whole milk or half and half*
sprinkle of ground cinnamon

DIRECTIONS

Add the water, honey and cinnamon sticks to a small saucepan. Set the pan over medium-high heat and cook, stirring frequently, until the honey has completely dissolved into the water. Let the mixture just come to a boil, then turn down the heat and let simmer gently for 5 minutes. Remove from the heat and stir in the vanilla extract.
Let the mixture cool completely then remove the cinnamon sticks (and discard).
Store the syrup in the refrigerator until ready to use.
TO SERVE:
Add some ice cubes to a serving glass. Pour in the cold brew coffee. Add in the desired amount of milk and honey cinnamon simple syrup, then mix to combine. Sprinkle the top with a touch of cinnamon. Serve immediately.

Baby Spinach and Dill Smoothie

Yield: 1

Ingredients

- ½ pear
- 1 cup frozen pineapple
- 1 cup chopped and seeded cucumber
- ¼ cup chopped fresh dill
- 1 cup baby spinach
- 1 small avocado
- 2 tablespoons lime juice
- 1-inch knob fresh gingerroot, peeled
- 3-4 ice cubes
- 1 tablespoon organic chia seeds
1 ¼ cup water

Directions

Place all ingredients, except for the ice and chia seeds, in a high speed blender and process until smooth and creamy. Add the ice and process again. Stir in chia seeds. Drink chilled.

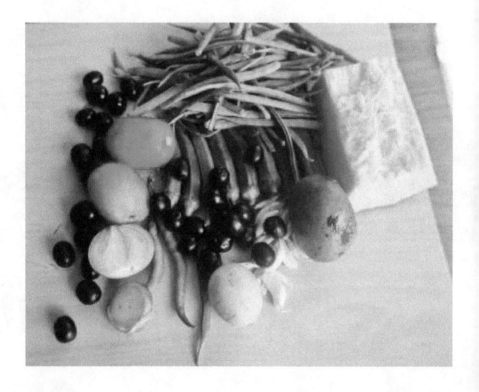